MAKING BEAUTY AND ORGANIC SKINCARE PRODUCTS FOR BEGINNERS

DIY Recipes, Natural Ingredients, Sustainable Techniques For Glowing Integument And Healthier Beauty Routines

ALFORD BARTELL

DISCLAIMER

The author of this book is not linked, associated, authorized, sponsored, or otherwise related to any corporation, business, or person mentioned in this book. This book was written based on the author's expertise, insight, and personal experiences. The material given is intended for educational and informative purposes only and should not be construed as professional advice. The author and publisher accept no responsibility or liability for any mistakes or omissions in the contents of this book. All thoughts stated are solely those of the author and do not represent the views of any organizations.

Table of Contents

ABOUT THIS BOOK

Making Beauty And Organic Skincare Products is a comprehensive guide designed to empower readers to create their own high-quality, organic skincare products from the comfort of their homes. This essential resource delves deeply into the world of organic skincare, offering both foundational knowledge and practical recipes to elevate your beauty routine with natural ingredients.

This book starts by introducing readers to the world of organic skincare, highlighting the numerous benefits of using natural ingredients over synthetic ones. It underscores the significance of understanding the organic skincare industry and addresses common myths that might deter individuals from exploring these products. The guide provides a clear pathway for beginners to embark on their DIY skincare journey, ensuring they have the knowledge to make informed choices about their skincare routines.

Understanding individual skin types and needs is crucial, and this guide expertly breaks down the characteristics of various skin types—dry, oily, combination, and sensitive. It offers insightful advice on identifying your skin type and tailoring products to meet specific needs. With a focus on solving common skin issues and the importance of patch testing, readers are equipped to create effective solutions for their unique skincare concerns.

This book also covers essential ingredients for organic skincare, detailing the benefits of carrier oils, essential oils, natural butter, and herbal infusions. It guides readers through selecting safe preservatives and emulsifiers, ensuring that their homemade products are both effective and safe.

For those new to DIY skincare, the guide provides a thorough overview of the basic equipment and tools required. It includes advice on must-have tools, safety precautions, and best practices for measuring, mixing, and storing products. This section ensures that readers can confidently create their skincare products while maintaining high standards of cleanliness and safety.

The guide offers practical recipes for a wide range of skincare products, including facial cleansers, toners, moisturizers, and serums. It explores various types of cleansers and toners and provides step-by-step instructions for crafting products suited to different skin types and concerns. For those interested in body care, it includes easy-to-follow recipes for lotions, scrubs, and balms. Additionally, this book addresses natural hair care solutions, featuring DIY recipes for shampoos and conditioners, and tips for maintaining healthy hair.

Packaging and labeling are crucial aspects of creating and selling skincare products. This guide emphasizes the importance of proper packaging, explores eco-friendly options, and offers advice on designing effective labels. It also covers legal requirements and marketing strategies, helping readers not only create but also successfully market their homemade products.

Finally, this book highlights the importance of sustainable and ethical practices in skincare. It discusses sourcing ethical ingredients, reducing waste, and supporting fair trade, encouraging readers to adopt environmentally friendly and socially responsible practices in their skincare routines.

Overall, Making Beauty And Organic Skincare Products is an invaluable resource for anyone interested in exploring the art of organic skincare. With its detailed instructions, practical tips, and ethical considerations, this guide empowers readers to create personalized, effective, and environmentally conscious beauty products.

CHAPTER ONE

Introduction To Organic Skincare

Definition And Benefits Of Organic Skincare

Organic skincare refers to the use of products made from natural ingredients that are cultivated without the use of synthetic chemicals, pesticides, or genetically modified organisms (GMOs). These products rely on ingredients sourced from organic farming practices, which emphasize the use of natural fertilizers and environmentally friendly methods. The primary benefit of organic skincare is its reduced risk of exposing the skin to potentially harmful chemicals. Unlike conventional skincare products that may contain artificial additives, preservatives, and synthetic fragrances, organic products aim to nourish the skin with ingredients that are as close to their natural state as possible.

In addition to being safer for the skin, organic skincare products are often more environmentally friendly. Organic farming practices help maintain soil health, reduce pollution, and promote biodiversity. For those with sensitive skin or allergies, organic skincare can offer a gentler alternative that minimizes irritation and adverse reactions. Many users also appreciate the ethical aspect of organic products, which often align with cruelty-free and fair-trade principles, supporting both animal welfare and fair labor practices.

Importance Of Natural Ingredients

Natural ingredients play a crucial role in organic skincare due to their inherent benefits for the skin. Unlike synthetic ingredients, which can sometimes cause allergic reactions or disrupt the skin's natural balance, natural ingredients tend to be more compatible with the body's processes. Ingredients like aloe vera, chamomile, and green tea are known for their soothing, anti-inflammatory, and antioxidant properties, respectively. These properties can help address various skin concerns, from dryness and redness to signs of aging.

When selecting natural ingredients, it's important to understand their specific benefits and how they interact with the skin. For instance, essential oils derived from plants not only add fragrance but also offer therapeutic benefits, such as calming or invigorating effects. Additionally, natural preservatives like vitamin E and rosemary extract can help extend the shelf life of skincare products without resorting to synthetic chemicals. By choosing natural ingredients, you are enhancing the efficacy and safety of your skincare routine, making it more aligned with holistic health practices.

Overview Of The Skincare Industry

The skincare industry is vast and continually evolving, encompassing a wide range of products designed to address various skin types and concerns. Traditional skincare products often rely on synthetic ingredients and complex formulations, which can sometimes make it challenging for consumers to discern what is truly beneficial for their skin. In recent years, there has been a significant shift towards organic and natural skincare as consumers become more informed about the potential risks associated with synthetic chemicals and express a growing preference for sustainable and ethical practices.

The rise of organic skincare has led to a broader range of products available on the market, from cleansers and moisturizers to serums and masks. This shift reflects a growing awareness of the impact that skincare products have not only on personal health but also on the environment. Many brands now emphasize transparency in their ingredient lists and production processes, allowing consumers to make more informed choices. Understanding this landscape helps consumers appreciate the value of organic skincare and encourages them to explore how they can create their products.

Common Myths About Organic Products

There are several myths surrounding organic skincare products that can create confusion for those new to the field. One common myth is that organic products are not as effective as their synthetic counterparts. In reality, many organic ingredients are rich in active compounds that can provide significant skincare benefits.

For example, organic honey has natural antibacterial properties, while organic rosehip oil is known for its regenerative effects on the skin.

Another myth is that organic products are always more expensive than conventional products. While some organic skincare items can be pricier due to the cost of sourcing high-quality ingredients and sustainable practices, making your organic skincare products can be a cost-effective alternative. By sourcing raw ingredients directly and learning to formulate your products, you can control both the cost and quality of your skincare routine.

A third myth is that organic skincare products have a shorter shelf life compared to synthetic products. While it's true that natural preservatives are used, many organic products can be stored effectively with proper handling and care.

Understanding how to properly store and preserve your homemade products can help maintain their efficacy and extend their shelf life.

Steps To Get Started In Making Your Products

Getting started with making your organic skincare products involves a few key steps that can simplify the process and ensure success. First, gather information about the ingredients you want to use and their benefits. This will help you create products that address specific skin concerns or needs. Researching common organic ingredients, such as shea butter, coconut oil, and essential oils, will give you a solid foundation for formulating your recipes.

Next, acquire high-quality, organic raw materials. Purchase these ingredients from reputable suppliers to ensure they are pure and free from contaminants. Some essential items you might need include carrier oils, essential oils, beeswax, and natural exfoliants. Investing in quality ingredients will enhance the effectiveness of your products and contribute to a more satisfying DIY experience.

After gathering your ingredients, begin with simple formulations such as facial cleansers or moisturizers. Start by following basic recipes and gradually experiment with variations as you become more comfortable with the process. It's important to maintain cleanliness and proper hygiene while making your products to avoid contamination.

Finally, store your homemade products in clean, airtight containers and label them with the date of creation. Keep them in a cool, dry place to extend their shelf life.

CHAPTER TWO

Understanding Skin Types And Needs

Different Skin Types (Dry, Oily, Combination, Sensitive)

Understanding the different skin types is crucial for creating effective beauty and skincare products. Each skin type has distinct characteristics and needs, so tailoring your products accordingly ensures better results and avoids potential irritation.

Dry Skin: This type is often characterized by a lack of moisture, leading to a rough texture, flakiness, and tightness. Dry skin may feel uncomfortable, especially in cold or windy conditions. To address dry skin, use ingredients that offer deep hydration and moisture retention, such as hyaluronic acid, glycerin, and natural oils like almond or jojoba oil. When formulating products for dry skin, focus on creating rich, emollient formulas that lock in moisture and prevent water loss.

Oily Skin: Oily skin is marked by excess sebum production, which can lead to a shiny appearance and frequent breakouts. This skin type often experiences enlarged pores and a greasy texture. To manage oily skin, opt for products that control oil production and balance the skin's natural oils. Ingredients such as salicylic acid, tea tree oil, and clay can help absorb excess oil and reduce shine. Formulations should be lightweight and non-comedogenic to avoid clogging pores.

Combination Skin: Combination skin features characteristics of both dry and oily skin, typically with an oily T-zone (forehead, nose, and chin) and dry or normal cheeks. Balancing products for combination skin requires addressing the varying needs of different areas. Use a combination of hydrating ingredients for dry patches and oil-control agents for the oily zones. Lightweight, balancing formulas are ideal for maintaining equilibrium across the face.

Sensitive Skin: Sensitive skin is prone to redness, irritation, and allergic reactions. It often reacts adversely to harsh ingredients or environmental factors. For sensitive skin, focus on gentle, soothing ingredients like chamomile, aloe vera, and calendula. Avoid products with synthetic fragrances, dyes, or alcohol. Formulations should be free from potential irritants and designed to calm and protect the skin.

Identifying Your Skin Type

Accurately identifying your skin type is the first step in creating effective skincare products. Start by cleansing your face with a gentle cleanser and wait for about an hour to observe how your skin behaves. During this time, avoid applying any products or touching your face.

Dry Skin: If your skin feels tight, rough, or flaky after cleansing, it is likely to dry. You might also notice dry patches or redness.

Oily Skin: If your skin appears shiny, especially in the T-zone, and feels greasy to the touch, you likely have oily skin. Look for enlarged pores and frequent breakouts as additional indicators.

Combination Skin: Combination skin can be identified if you notice a mix of both oily and dry areas. For instance, your T-zone may appear greasy while your cheeks feel dry or normal.

Sensitive Skin: Sensitive skin often reacts to environmental changes or skincare products with redness, itching, or burning. If you experience frequent irritation, you might have sensitive skin.

To confirm your skin type, you can use a skin analysis tool or consult with a dermatologist. Knowing your skin type helps in selecting the right ingredients and formulations for your homemade skincare products.

Tailoring Products To Skin Needs

Once you've identified your skin type, tailoring your skincare products to meet your specific needs is essential. This ensures that your products are effective and beneficial for your skin.

For Dry Skin: Choose hydrating and nourishing ingredients that replenish moisture. Incorporate oils, butter, and humectants into your formulations. Create rich creams or serums that provide long-lasting hydration and prevent moisture loss.

For Oily Skin: Opt for lightweight, oil-free ingredients that control excess sebum. Use astringents and mattifying agents to manage oil production. Formulate gels or foaming cleansers that help balance oil levels without over-drying the skin.

For Combination Skin: Create products that address both oily and dry areas. Formulate balanced moisturizers that hydrate without being greasy, and use exfoliants that can handle both dry patches and oily zones.

For Sensitive Skin: Focus on calming and soothing ingredients. Formulate products that are hypoallergenic and free from potential irritants. Opt for non-fragranced, gentle formulations that reduce the risk of sensitivity.

Tailoring your products involves selecting the right combination of ingredients that address the specific needs of your skin type, ensuring your skincare routine is effective and comfortable.

Common Skin Issues And Solutions

Various skin issues can arise, and understanding how to address them effectively is vital for successful skincare. Here are some common issues and their solutions:

Acne: Acne can result from excess oil, clogged pores, and bacteria. Use products with salicylic acid, benzoyl peroxide, or tea tree oil to help reduce breakouts. Incorporate exfoliating ingredients to clear dead skin cells and prevent pore clogging.

Hyperpigmentation: Dark spots or uneven skin tone can be caused by sun exposure or acne scars. Use ingredients like vitamin C, niacinamide, and alpha hydroxy acids (AHAs) to brighten the skin and even out pigmentation.

Redness and Irritation: Redness and irritation often occur in sensitive skin. Use soothing ingredients such as aloe vera, chamomile, and green tea. Avoid products with alcohol, fragrances, or harsh chemicals that can exacerbate these issues.

Dryness and Flakiness: Dryness and flakiness can be managed by using hydrating and emollient ingredients like hyaluronic acid, glycerin, and shea butter. Regular exfoliation with mild scrubs or chemical exfoliants can also help remove dead skin cells and improve moisture absorption.

By addressing these common issues with targeted ingredients, you can effectively manage and improve your skin's overall health and appearance.

Importance Of Patch Testing

Patch testing is a crucial step in ensuring that your homemade skincare products are safe and suitable for your skin. It helps to identify any potential allergic reactions or irritations before using a product more extensively.

How to Perform a Patch Test: Apply a small amount of the product to a discreet area of skin, such as the inside of your wrist or behind your ear. Cover the area with a bandage or adhesive strip and leave it for 24 to 48 hours. Observe for any signs of redness, itching, swelling, or irritation. If any adverse reactions occur, discontinue the use of the product.

Why Patch Testing is Important: Patch testing helps prevent unwanted reactions and ensures that the ingredients in your product are compatible with your skin.

It is especially important when using new or unfamiliar ingredients.

When to Patch Test: Always perform a patch test when trying new ingredients or formulations, even if the ingredients are commonly used. This precaution helps avoid unexpected allergic reactions and ensures the safety of your skincare products.

By incorporating patch testing into your skincare routine, you can confidently use homemade products without the risk of irritation or adverse reactions.

CHAPTER THREE

Essential Ingredients For Organic Skincare

Carrier Oils And Their Benefits

Carrier oils are fundamental in organic skincare as they dilute essential oils and deliver their benefits to the skin. These oils are extracted from the seeds, nuts, or kernels of plants, and each offers unique properties that can enhance your skincare routine. To make the most of carrier oils, it's essential to understand their different benefits and how to choose the right one for your skin type.

Common Carrier Oils

1.   **Jojoba Oil:** Jojoba oil closely resembles the skin's natural sebum, making it an excellent

choice for balancing oil production and moisturizing. It is non-comedogenic, meaning it won't clog pores, and is suitable for all skin types, including sensitive skin. To use, simply apply a few drops directly to the skin or mix it into your homemade moisturizer or serum.

2.   **Argan Oil:** Rich in vitamin E and essential fatty acids, argan oil is known for its hydrating and anti-aging properties. It helps to restore the skin's elasticity and reduce the appearance of fine lines. To incorporate argan oil into your routine, you can use it as a daily moisturizer or add it to facial masks and creams.

3.   **Rosehip Seed Oil:** This oil is renowned for its regenerative properties, making it ideal for treating scars, hyperpigmentation, and signs of aging. It's high in essential fatty acids and vitamins A and C, which promote skin cell regeneration.

To use, apply a few drops to your face or mix it with other carrier oils for a nourishing serum.

How to Use Carrier Oils

Carrier oils can be used alone or blended with other oils to suit your skin's needs. When creating your skincare products, start with a base of one or two carrier oils. For instance, blend jojoba oil with argan oil to create a balanced moisturizer that hydrates and soothes. Use a ratio of about 70% carrier oil to 30% essential oil in your blends. Always perform a patch test before applying any new oil to your skin to ensure there are no adverse reactions.

Essential Oils And Their Properties

Essential oils are concentrated plant extracts that provide therapeutic benefits for the skin. Each essential oil has its unique properties, such as antibacterial, anti-inflammatory, or soothing effects, which can be harnessed in organic skincare formulations. Understanding these properties allows you to tailor your products to address specific skin concerns.

1.   **Lavender Oil:** Known for its calming and healing properties, lavender oil is excellent for soothing irritated skin and reducing redness. It also promotes relaxation and can be added to a nighttime skincare routine to improve sleep quality. To use, add a few drops to a diffuser or mix with carrier oil for topical application.

2.   **Tea Tree Oil:** Tea tree oil has powerful antibacterial and antifungal properties, making it ideal for treating acne-prone skin. It helps to reduce inflammation and clear blemishes. Dilute tea tree oil with a carrier oil before applying it

directly to the affected areas of the skin to prevent irritation.

3. **Chamomile Oil:** This oil is celebrated for its anti-inflammatory and soothing effects, making it beneficial for sensitive or inflamed skin. It helps to calm redness and irritation. Use chamomile oil in facial creams or masks to soothe and heal the skin.

How to Incorporate Essential Oils

To incorporate essential oils into your skincare routine, always dilute them with carrier oils to avoid skin irritation. Use about 5-10 drops of essential oil per ounce of carrier oil or skincare product. Add essential oils to homemade lotions, face masks, or serums, mixing well to ensure even distribution. Store essential oil blends in dark glass bottles to preserve their potency.

Natural Butters (Shea, Cocoa, Mango)

Natural butter are rich, creamy substance derived from the seeds or fruits of plants. They are known for their emollient properties, making them excellent for moisturizing and nourishing the skin. Each type of butter has unique benefits that can enhance your skincare formulations.

Shea Butter

Shea butter is renowned for its deep moisturizing and healing properties. It is rich in vitamins A and E, which help to soothe and protect the skin. Shea butter is excellent for treating dry skin, eczema, and minor burns. To use shea butter, melt it in a double boiler, and mix it with other oils or essential oils before applying it to the skin. It can also be whipped into a light, airy body butter for a luxurious texture.

Cocoa Butter

Cocoa butter is known for its ability to improve skin elasticity and reduce the appearance of stretch marks. It has a rich, creamy texture that helps to lock in moisture and smooth the skin. Cocoa butter is best used in body lotions and balms. Melt cocoa butter gently and combine it with other carrier oils and essential oils to create a hydrating body lotion.

Mango Butter

Mango butter is a lesser-known butter that is high in vitamins A and C, making it ideal for rejuvenating and brightening the skin. It has a lighter texture compared to shea and cocoa butter, making it suitable for use in facial creams. Mango butter can be melted and mixed with other butter or oils to create a nourishing face cream or body butter.

Herbal Infusions And Extracts

Herbal infusions and extracts are created by soaking herbs in carrier oils or solvents to extract their beneficial compounds. These infusions can be used to enhance the therapeutic properties of your skincare products. Understanding how to make and use these extracts can elevate your organic skincare formulations.

Making Herbal Infusions

To make a herbal infusion, start by selecting dried herbs such as chamomile, calendula, or lavender. Place the herbs in a clean glass jar and cover them with carrier oil, such as jojoba or olive oil. Seal the jar and let it sit in a warm, sunny place for 2-4 weeks, shaking it occasionally. Strain the oil through a fine mesh sieve or cheesecloth into a clean bottle.

This infused oil can be used in creams, lotions, and balms for added herbal benefits.

Preparing Herbal Extracts

Herbal extracts are concentrated solutions made by soaking herbs in alcohol or glycerin. To make a glycerin extract, mix dried herbs with vegetable glycerin and water in a glass jar. Let the mixture sit for several weeks, shaking it daily. Strain the extract through a fine mesh sieve or cheesecloth. Glycerin extracts are less potent than alcohol-based extracts but are suitable for those with sensitive skin.

Using Herbal Infusions and Extracts

Incorporate herbal infusions and extracts into your skincare products by adding them to creams, serums, or masks. Use herbal infusions at a concentration of 10-20% in your formulations.

For extracts, follow the recommended usage guidelines on the product label. These additions can enhance the soothing, anti-inflammatory, or antimicrobial properties of your skincare products.

Safe Preservatives And Emulsifiers

Preservatives and emulsifiers are essential for extending the shelf life and stability of homemade skincare products. Natural preservatives help prevent microbial growth, while emulsifiers keep oil and water from separating. Using the right preservatives and emulsifiers ensures that your products remain safe and effective.

Natural Preservatives

1.   **Vitamin E:** Vitamin E is a natural antioxidant that helps prevent oils from going rancid.

It also provides additional skin benefits, such as moisturizing and protecting against oxidative stress. To use, add a few drops of vitamin E oil to your homemade creams and lotions.

2.   **Rosemary Extract:** Rosemary extract has natural antimicrobial properties that help to preserve the freshness of your skincare products. It also acts as an antioxidant. Use rosemary extract at a concentration of 0.5-1% in your formulations to help extend shelf life.

Emulsifiers

1.   **Beeswax:** Beeswax is a natural emulsifier that helps to bind oil and water in skincare products. It also provides a protective barrier on the skin. To use, melt beeswax with carrier oils and blend with water or hydrosols to create a stable emulsion.

2.   **Lecithin:** Lecithin is derived from soy or sunflower and acts as a gentle emulsifier. It helps to mix oil and water and can improve the texture of your products. Use lecithin in a concentration of 1-3% in your formulations.

How to Use Preservatives and Emulsifiers

When creating your skin care products, incorporate preservatives and emulsifiers according to their recommended usage rates. For example, add vitamin E or rosemary extract to your formulations to protect against spoilage. Combine beeswax or lecithin with your oils and water to create stable emulsions. Always store your products in clean, airtight containers to maintain their effectiveness and safety.

CHAPTER FOUR

Basic Equipment And Tools

Must-Have Tools For Beginners

When starting in the world of beauty and organic skincare product making, having the right tools is essential to ensure a smooth and successful process. For beginners, the basic toolkit should include a few fundamental items:

1. **Mixing Bowls:** Opt for glass or stainless steel mixing bowls, as these materials are non-reactive and won't interfere with the ingredients. Small to medium-sized bowls are ideal for various formulations, from face masks to serums.

2. **Spatulas and Spoons:** Silicone spatulas and stainless steel spoons are perfect for stirring and transferring ingredients.

Silicone is particularly useful for scraping down the sides of bowls to ensure no ingredient is left behind.

3.   **Measuring Cups and Spoons:** Accurate measurements are crucial in skincare formulations. Invest in a set of measuring cups (both dry and liquid) and measuring spoons to ensure precise quantities of ingredients.

4.   **Whisks and Blenders:** A hand whisk or small electric mixer is useful for blending ingredients smoothly. For more advanced formulations, a stick blender can help achieve a consistent texture in creams and emulsions.

These tools are the foundation of your skincare-making kit. They are versatile and will serve you well across various recipes and formulations.

Safety is paramount when crafting skincare products, especially when dealing with essential oils, preservatives, and other potentially irritating ingredients. Here's how to ensure a safe environment:

1.   **Gloves:** Wear disposable gloves to protect your hands from direct contact with ingredients, especially those that may irritate. Gloves also help maintain hygiene and prevent contamination of your products.

2.   **Safety Goggles:** Safety goggles are a must if you're working with strong essential oils or any ingredients that could splash. They protect your eyes from accidental exposure and potential irritation.

3.   **Face Masks:** To avoid inhaling dust or fumes from certain ingredients, use a face mask.

This is particularly important when working with powdered ingredients or during the mixing of volatile substances.

4.   **Aprons:** Protect your clothing and skin from spills and splashes with a lab apron or a dedicated apron for skincare-making. It's an easy way to maintain a clean workspace.

Adhering to these safety measures will help you create products without risking your health or safety.

Measuring And Mixing Tools

Accurate measurement and proper mixing are critical for the effectiveness and stability of skincare products. Here's a breakdown of how to effectively use these tools:

1.   **Digital Scale:** A digital scale is essential for precise measurement of both liquids and solids.

It ensures that you use the exact amount of each ingredient, which is crucial for achieving consistent results.

2.   **Measuring Spoons and Cups:** Use these for smaller quantities and ensure they are calibrated. For instance, measuring spoons come in different sizes (teaspoons and tablespoons), and using the right size helps in maintaining recipe accuracy.

3.   **Mixing Tools:** Utilize whisks, spatulas, and blenders according to the recipe. For example, whisking is ideal for emulsifying oils and water, while spatulas are great for mixing thick substances like butter or creams.

4.   **Thermometers:** Some skincare recipes require specific temperatures for melting or combining ingredients. A good thermometer helps you monitor and maintain the correct temperature, ensuring ingredient integrity.

By following these guidelines, you can measure and mix your ingredients with precision, resulting in well-balanced and effective skincare products.

Storage Containers And Labeling

Proper storage and labeling are crucial to ensure the longevity and safety of your skincare products. Here's how to manage this effectively:

1.   **Containers:** Use airtight containers to prevent contamination and preserve the integrity of your products. Glass jars are excellent for creams and serums, while plastic bottles with pumps are ideal for liquid products. Ensure the containers are clean and dry before use.

2.   **Labels:** Clearly label your products with the name, date of creation, and any special instructions or ingredients. This not only helps in

tracking the freshness but also aids in avoiding confusion and ensures proper use.

3.   **Storage Conditions:** Store your products in a cool, dark place to extend their shelf life. Avoid exposure to heat and sunlight, which can degrade ingredients and reduce the effectiveness of your products.

4.   **Shelf Life Monitoring:** Regularly check your products for any changes in color, smell, or texture. Discard any products that show signs of spoilage or degradation to avoid potential adverse effects.

By properly storing and labeling your products, you ensure their safety and effectiveness for the intended period.

Maintaining clean and well-maintained tools is essential for the quality and safety of your skincare products. Here's a practical approach to cleaning and maintaining your tools:

1.   **Routine Cleaning:** Wash your mixing bowls, spoons, and spatulas with warm, soapy water after each use. Rinse thoroughly to remove any soap residue. For tools that come into contact with oils, a mixture of baking soda and water can help remove grease.

2.   **Sanitization:** For a deeper clean, sanitize your tools with a solution of 70% isopropyl alcohol. This helps eliminate any bacteria or residue that might be left behind.

3.   **Drying:** Allow all tools to air dry completely before storing them.

This prevents moisture from causing mold or mildew growth. Store tools in a clean, dry place.

4.   **Tool Inspection:** Regularly inspect your tools for any signs of wear or damage. Replace any tools that are cracked or chipped, as they can harbor bacteria or affect the quality of your formulations.

By keeping your tools clean and in good condition, you ensure a safer and more efficient skincare-making process.

CHAPTER FIVE

Making Organic Facial Cleansers

Types Of Cleansers

Oil-Based Cleansers

Oil-based cleansers are ideal for removing makeup and impurities without stripping the skin of its natural oils. They work on the principle that "like dissolves like"—the oil in the cleanser binds with the oil-based impurities on your skin, allowing them to be washed away easily. To make a basic oil-based cleanser, mix equal parts of a carrier oil such as sweet almond oil or jojoba oil with a small amount of castor oil. The castor oil helps to emulsify the oils and provides a deeper cleanse. Simply massage the mixture onto your dry face, and then rinse with warm water. For a more luxurious feel, you can add a few drops of essential oils like lavender or chamomile for additional soothing properties.

Foaming Cleansers

Foaming cleansers are great for those who prefer a lathering experience. They are effective at removing excess oil and dirt. To create a basic foaming cleanser, blend one tablespoon of liquid Castile soap with one tablespoon of water and a few drops of essential oil. Pour the mixture into a foaming pump bottle. The Castile soap will create a gentle foam that cleanses the skin, while the essential oils can be tailored to your skin type (e.g., tea tree oil for acne-prone skin). Shake the bottle before each use and pump a small amount onto your wet face, massaging gently before rinsing off with lukewarm water.

Micellar water is a versatile and gentle option for cleansing. It contains tiny micelles that attract dirt and oil, making it easy to remove them without rinsing. To make micellar water, mix one cup of distilled water with two tablespoons of witch hazel and one teaspoon of mild liquid Castile soap. Add a few drops of essential oil, such as rose or chamomile, for added benefits. Store the mixture in a clean bottle and shake well before use. Apply it to a cotton pad and gently wipe over your face. It's perfect for a quick cleanse or removing makeup without the need for rinsing.

Basic Recipes For Different Skin Types

Dry Skin

For dry skin, a hydrating and soothing cleanser is key. Combine one-quarter cup of coconut oil with one-quarter cup of honey. Coconut oil is moisturizing, while honey has antibacterial and humectant properties that help retain moisture. Gently massage the mixture onto your face, then wipe off with a warm, damp cloth. This cleanser helps to nourish and hydrate the skin while cleansing away impurities.

Oily Skin

For oily skin, a balancing and deep-cleansing recipe is effective. Mix one-quarter cup of aloe vera gel with two tablespoons of witch hazel and one tablespoon of jojoba oil. Aloe vera helps to soothe and control oil production, witch hazel acts as an astringent, and jojoba oil helps to regulate sebum levels. Apply the mixture to your face, massage gently, and rinse with cool water. This combination helps to cleanse the skin thoroughly while controlling excess oil.

Sensitive Skin

Sensitive skin requires a gentle and calming cleanser. Combine one-quarter cup of unsweetened yogurt with one tablespoon of honey and a few drops of chamomile essential oil. Yogurt is soothing and contains lactic acid to gently exfoliate, while honey hydrates and chamomile calms the skin. Apply the mixture to your face, leave it on for a few minutes to allow the ingredients to work, then rinse with lukewarm water. This recipe helps to cleanse without irritating.

Customizing With Essential Oils

Essential oils can be added to any facial cleanser recipe to address specific skin concerns. For acne-prone skin, consider adding a few drops of tea tree oil or lavender oil, known for their antibacterial properties. For dry skin, rose or geranium essential oils can provide additional hydration and soothing effects. Always dilute essential oils properly (usually 2-3 drops per tablespoon of carrier or base ingredient) to avoid skin irritation. Perform a patch test before using any new essential oil in your cleanser to ensure you do not have an adverse reaction.

Proper Usage And Storage

When using homemade organic facial cleansers, it's important to follow proper application and storage methods. For most cleansers, apply a small amount to your damp face, massage gently in circular motions, and rinse thoroughly with lukewarm water. Be sure to follow up with a moisturizer suited to your skin type to lock in hydration.

Store your homemade cleansers in clean, airtight containers to extend their shelf life. For oil-based and foaming cleansers, use dark glass bottles to protect the ingredients from light, which can cause degradation. Micellar water and other liquid cleansers should be stored in cool, dry places and used within a few weeks to ensure freshness.

Troubleshooting Common Issues

Cleansers Not Removing Makeup Effectively

If your cleanser isn't removing makeup thoroughly, it may be too gentle or not formulated correctly.

Try adding a small amount of castor oil to your oil-based cleanser to enhance its emulsifying properties. Alternatively, use a two-step cleansing method: first with an oil-based cleanser to break down makeup, followed by a foaming or micellar cleanser for a deep clean.

Cleansers Causing Dryness or Irritation

If you experience dryness or irritation, it may be due to overly harsh ingredients or an imbalance in the formula. Reduce the amount of essential oils or avoid those known for their drying effects. Opt for more soothing ingredients like aloe vera or honey, and ensure your cleanser is well-formulated for your skin type. Consider using the cleanser less frequently or switch to a more hydrating recipe.

Cleansers Separating or Changing Texture

If your cleanser separates or changes texture, it may be due to improper mixing or ingredient instability.

Shake or stir the cleanser before each use to ensure a consistent texture. For oil-based and foaming cleansers, ensure that the oils and other components are well-blended. Store the cleanser in a stable, cool environment to prevent separation and degradation.

CHAPTER SIX

Crafting Natural Toners

Benefits Of Using Toners

Toners are essential in skincare routines for a variety of reasons. They help to restore the skin's natural pH balance after cleansing, which is crucial because many cleansers can be alkaline and disrupt the skin's acidity. This balance is important for maintaining healthy skin and can help to prevent issues such as dryness and irritation.

In addition to balancing pH, toners can help remove any residual impurities left after cleansing. This includes traces of dirt, oil, and makeup that might clog pores and lead to breakouts.

By ensuring that your skin is thoroughly clean, toners prepare the skin for subsequent skincare products, allowing them to penetrate more effectively.

Toners can also provide a boost of hydration, which is beneficial for maintaining the skin's moisture levels and elasticity. Many toners contain ingredients that soothe and calm the skin, reducing redness and inflammation. This can be particularly useful for individuals with sensitive or acne-prone skin.

Ingredients For Hydrating And Balancing Toners

When crafting natural toners, selecting the right ingredients is crucial. Hydrating ingredients like rose water and aloe vera gel are excellent choices. Rose water is known for its soothing properties and ability to reduce redness and irritation.

Aloe vera gel provides deep hydration and helps to heal and soothe the skin.

Another beneficial ingredient is witch hazel, which acts as a natural astringent. It helps to tighten pores and reduce excess oil without stripping the skin of its natural moisture. For a balancing toner, consider adding green tea extract, which is rich in antioxidants and can help to reduce inflammation and protect the skin from environmental damage.

Essential oils can also be used to enhance the benefits of your toner. Lavender oil has calming properties, while tea tree oil is known for its antibacterial benefits. It's important to use essential oils in moderation and always dilute them properly, as they can be potent and may cause irritation if used in high concentrations.

1. Hydrating Rose Water Toner

Ingredients:

1 cup rose water

1 tablespoon aloe vera gel

5 drops of lavender essential oil

Instructions:

In a clean spray bottle, combine the rose water and aloe vera gel.

Add the lavender essential oil and shake well to mix.

To use, mist the toner over your face after cleansing. Allow it to absorb before applying other skincare products.

2. Balancing Witch Hazel Toner

Ingredients:

1/2 cup witch hazel

1/2 cup distilled water

1 tablespoon green tea extract

3 drops of tea tree essential oil

Instructions:

Mix the witch hazel and distilled water in a clean bottle.

Add the green tea extract and tea tree oil, then shake well.

Apply with a cotton pad to the face and neck, avoiding the eye area. This toner can help control oil and reduce acne.

3. Soothing Aloe and Chamomile Toner

Ingredients:

1/2 cup aloe vera juice

1/2 cup chamomile tea (cooled)

1 tablespoon honey

Instructions:

Brew chamomile tea and let it cool completely.

In a bottle, combine aloe vera juice and cooled chamomile tea.

Stir in the honey until fully dissolved.

Apply with a cotton pad to soothe and hydrate the skin.

Application Techniques

When applying toners, it's essential to use proper techniques to maximize their effectiveness. Start by cleansing your face thoroughly to remove any makeup or impurities. After cleansing, apply the toner using a cotton pad or by misting it directly onto your face.

For cotton pad application, gently swipe the pad over your skin in upward, and outward motions. This helps to avoid dragging or irritating the skin. If you're using a spray bottle, hold it about 6-8 inches from your face and mist the toner evenly. Allow it to dry naturally before proceeding with your moisturizer or other skincare products.

Avoid applying toner too close to the eyes, as the delicate skin around this area can be sensitive. If using essential oils, ensure they are diluted properly to prevent irritation. Using toners in the morning and evening can help maintain balanced and hydrated skin throughout the day and night.

Storing And Preserving Homemade Toners

To ensure your homemade toners remain effective and safe, proper storage is key. Use clean, airtight containers to prevent contamination. Glass bottles are ideal, as they do not react with the ingredients and are easier to clean.

Store your toner in a cool, dark place to extend its shelf life. Avoid exposing it to direct sunlight or high temperatures, which can degrade the ingredients. Most homemade toners can be stored for up to 2-4 weeks, depending on the ingredients used. Always check for any changes in smell or appearance, which could indicate spoilage.

For added freshness, you can store your toner in the refrigerator. This not only extends its shelf life but also provides a refreshing, cooling sensation upon application. Remember to label your toner with the date it was made to keep track of its freshness and to ensure you use it within the recommended time frame.

CHAPTER SEVEN

Formulating Moisturizers And Serums

Difference Between Moisturizers And Serums

Moisturizers and serums are both essential components of a skincare routine but serve distinct functions. Moisturizers are designed to hydrate and lock in moisture, forming a barrier to prevent water loss. They typically contain occlusive agents like oils or butter that create a protective layer on the skin. These products are usually heavier and provide lasting hydration, making them ideal for daily use to maintain skin softness and prevent dryness.

Serums, on the other hand, are lightweight, concentrated treatments designed to target specific skin concerns.

They often contain higher concentrations of active ingredients such as vitamins, antioxidants, and peptides, which can penetrate deeper into the skin. Serums are used to address issues like aging, pigmentation, and uneven skin tone. Because they are more fluid and absorb quickly, serums are generally applied before moisturizers to enhance their effectiveness.

Understanding the difference between these two types of products helps in selecting the right ones for your skincare needs. While moisturizers provide a protective layer to keep skin hydrated, serums deliver potent ingredients that address targeted concerns. For optimal results, it's essential to incorporate both into your skincare regimen, using serums to treat specific issues and moisturizers to maintain overall skin health.

Key Ingredients For Hydration And Anti-Aging

When formulating your moisturizers and serums, it's crucial to choose ingredients that effectively address hydration and anti-aging. For hydration, look for ingredients like hyaluronic acid, glycerin, and aloe vera. Hyaluronic acid is known for its ability to hold moisture in the skin, making it a powerful hydrator. Glycerin attracts water from the environment and helps retain it in the skin, while aloe vera soothes and adds moisture.

Anti-aging ingredients include retinoids, vitamin C, and peptides. Retinoids, derived from vitamin A, help stimulate collagen production and improve skin texture. Vitamin C is a potent antioxidant that brightens the skin and reduces the appearance of dark spots. Peptides are small proteins that support the skin's barrier function and promote elasticity.

Combining these ingredients can yield a powerful skincare product. For instance, a serum with hyaluronic acid and vitamin C can provide both hydration and anti-aging benefits, while a moisturizer containing peptides and glycerin can improve skin firmness and retain moisture. By selecting the right ingredients, you can tailor your products to meet your specific skin needs and achieve noticeable results.

Simple Recipes For Various Skin Types

Creating your skincare products can be both fun and rewarding. Here are some simple recipes for moisturizers and serums suited to different skin types:

For Dry Skin:

1.   Hydrating Moisturizer:

2 tbsp shea butter

1 tbsp coconut oil

1 tbsp almond oil

5 drops of lavender essential oil

Melt the shea butter and coconut oil in a double boiler. Remove from heat and stir in almond oil and lavender essential oil. Allow the mixture to cool and solidify before use. This rich, nourishing moisturizer will leave dry skin feeling soft and hydrated.

2.   Soothing Serum:

1 tbsp rosehip oil

1 tbsp argan oil

5 drops of chamomile essential oil

Combine rosehip oil and argan oil in a small dropper bottle. Add chamomile essential oil and shake well. Apply a few drops to the face before moisturizing to soothe and hydrate dry skin.

For Oily Skin:

1.   Lightweight Moisturizer:

1 tbsp aloe vera gel

1 tbsp jojoba oil

5 drops of tea tree oil

Mix aloe vera gel and jojoba oil in a bowl. Add tea tree oil and stir thoroughly. Apply a thin layer to the face to balance oil production and provide hydration without clogging pores.

2.   Refreshing Serum:

1 tbsp witch hazel

1 tbsp rosewater

5 drops peppermint essential oil

Combine witch hazel and rosewater in a small spray bottle. Add peppermint essential oil and shake well. Spritz onto the face after cleansing to refresh and control oiliness.

For Sensitive Skin:

1.   Gentle Moisturizer:

2 tbsp shea butter

1 tbsp calendula oil

5 drops of frankincense essential oil

Melt shea butter and mix with calendula oil. Add frankincense essential oil and blend well. This gentle moisturizer helps soothe and calm sensitive skin while providing necessary hydration.

2.   Calming Serum:

1 tbsp chamomile oil

1 tbsp rosehip oil

5 drops of geranium essential oil

Mix chamomile oil and rosehip oil in a dropper bottle. Add geranium essential oil and shake. Apply a few drops to the skin to calm irritation and reduce redness.

Layering Techniques For Maximum Benefits

To achieve the best results from your moisturizers and serums, it's important to layer them correctly. Start with a clean, toned face to ensure that your skin is ready to absorb the products. Begin with your serum, as it contains concentrated active ingredients that need to penetrate deeply. Apply a few drops and gently press into the skin, focusing on areas that need the most attention.

Allow the serum to absorb fully before applying your moisturizer. This step is crucial as it ensures that the active ingredients from the serum are fully absorbed and that the moisturizer can form a barrier to lock in those benefits. Apply the moisturizer evenly across your face and neck, using upward strokes to promote circulation and help the product penetrate better.

Incorporating both products into your routine can maximize their effectiveness. For daytime use, consider using a lightweight serum and a non-greasy moisturizer to avoid feeling too heavy. At night, you can use a richer serum and a more hydrating moisturizer to allow your skin to repair and rejuvenate while you sleep. By following these layering techniques, you can enhance the efficacy of both your moisturizers and serums.

Packaging And Storage Tips

Proper packaging and storage are vital for maintaining the efficacy and longevity of your homemade skincare products.

Use airtight containers to prevent contamination and oxidation, which can degrade the quality of your ingredients. Glass jars or bottles with pump dispensers are ideal as they help protect the product from exposure to air and light.

Store your products in a cool, dry place away from direct sunlight to prevent them from breaking down. For items that contain ingredients prone to spoilage, like oils or natural extracts, refrigeration can help extend their shelf life. However, ensure that the container is properly sealed to avoid moisture accumulation inside.

Label your products with the date of creation and any special instructions for use. This practice helps you keep track of freshness and ensures that you use the products within their optimal time frame. Regularly check for any changes in texture, color, or smell, which can indicate that the product has gone bad.

CHAPTER EIGHT

Creating Body Care Products

Types Of Body Care Products

When it comes to body care, several essential products can be made at home with simple ingredients. Among these, lotions, scrubs, and balms are fundamental for maintaining healthy and radiant skin.

Body Lotions: Body lotions are designed to hydrate and soothe the skin. They typically consist of a blend of oils, butter, and water, which help lock in moisture and keep the skin soft. A basic lotion can be made by combining a carrier oil (like coconut or almond oil) with butter (such as shea or cocoa butter) and an emulsifying agent to blend the oil and water phases.

Body Scrubs: Scrubs are exfoliating products that help remove dead skin cells, revealing smoother and brighter skin. They usually contain a scrub agent, like sugar or salt, mixed with an oil or gel base. The scrub agent physically sloughs off dead skin cells, while the oil or gel moisturizes the skin.

Body Balms: Balms are thicker than lotions and are used for targeted areas that need extra moisture or relief. They often include a combination of oils, butter, beeswax, or another thickening agent to create a more solid consistency. Body balms are great for dry patches, elbows, knees, and heels.

Benefits Of Body Care Routines

Incorporating a regular body care routine can significantly enhance your skin's health and appearance.

Hydration: Daily application of body lotion ensures your skin remains hydrated and elastic. Hydrated skin is less prone to dryness, flakiness, and cracking, which can be particularly beneficial in harsh weather conditions.

Exfoliation: Regular use of body scrubs helps to remove dead skin cells, preventing clogged pores and promoting new cell growth. Exfoliation also improves the absorption of moisturizers and enhances the overall texture of the skin.

Healing and Protection: Body balms provide a protective layer on the skin, helping to soothe and heal areas prone to dryness or irritation. They are especially useful for areas that need a bit more attention, offering concentrated relief and protection.

Easy Recipes For Body Lotions And Scrubs

Basic Body Lotion Recipe:

1.   Ingredients:

1/2 cup coconut oil

1/4 cup shea butter

1/4 cup almond oil

1 teaspoon beeswax pellets (for thicker consistency)

Optional: a few drops of essential oil for fragrance

2.   Instructions:

Melt the coconut oil, shea butter, and beeswax together in a double boiler until fully combined.

Remove from heat and stir in the almond oil and essential oil.

Pour the mixture into a clean container and allow it to cool and solidify. Stir occasionally during the cooling process to maintain a smooth texture.

Simple Sugar Body Scrub Recipe:

1.   Ingredients:

1/2 cup granulated sugar

1/4 cup coconut oil

1/4 cup honey

Optional: 1 teaspoon of your favorite essential oil

2.   Instructions:

In a mixing bowl, combine the sugar, coconut oil, and honey until well blended.

Add essential oil if using, and mix thoroughly.

Transfer the scrub into a jar with a tight-fitting lid. Use it in the shower, gently massaging it into the skin to exfoliate and hydrate.

Incorporating Exfoliants And Moisturizers

Choosing Exfoliants: Exfoliants can be physical or chemical. Physical exfoliants include sugar, salt, or coffee grounds, which physically scrub away dead skin. Chemical exfoliants, like alpha hydroxy acids (AHAs) or beta hydroxy acids (BHAs), break down dead skin cells at a cellular level. For a basic at-home scrub, physical exfoliants are easy to use and effective.

Selecting Moisturizers: Moisturizers help to lock in hydration and protect the skin barrier. When choosing ingredients, consider using emollients (like oils and butter) that help to soften the skin and occlusives (like beeswax) that form a barrier to prevent moisture loss.

Application Tips:

Apply exfoliants in a circular motion to avoid skin irritation.

Use moisturizers after exfoliation to seal in moisture and keep the skin smooth.

For best results, exfoliate 1-2 times a week and moisturize daily.

Preserving And Storing Body Care Products

Preservation Techniques: Homemade body care products lack preservatives found in commercial products, so it's important to take steps to prevent spoilage. Use clean utensils and containers to avoid contamination. Adding a few drops of vitamin E oil can also help extend the shelf life of your products by acting as a natural preservative.

Storage Recommendations: Store your products in airtight containers to prevent exposure to air and moisture, which can lead to spoilage. Keep them in a cool, dark place, away from direct sunlight. Body lotions and balms can generally be stored for up to six months, while scrubs should be used within three months for optimal freshness.

Batch Size: If you're new to making body care products, start with small batches to test out your recipes and ensure they meet your needs. This will help you manage inventory and reduce waste. As you become more comfortable, you can scale up the quantities as needed.

By following these guidelines, you can create effective and enjoyable body care products right at home, ensuring your skincare routine is both natural and personalized.

CHAPTER NINE

Natural Hair Care Solutions

Understanding Hair Types And Needs

Understanding your hair type is the cornerstone of effective natural hair care. Hair types vary from straight to wavy, curly, and coily, and each type has its own unique needs and characteristics. For example, straight hair often requires less moisture compared to curly hair, which can be prone to dryness. To identify your hair type, observe its natural texture when it's clean and dry. Consider factors like how your hair holds curls or its reaction to humidity.

Additionally, understanding your hair's porosity—how well it absorbs and retains moisture—is crucial.

Hair with high porosity absorbs moisture quickly but loses it just as fast, whereas low-porosity hair takes longer to absorb moisture but retains it well. Conduct a simple porosity test by placing a strand of your hair in a glass of water. If it sinks quickly, you have high-porosity hair; if it floats or sinks slowly, your hair has low porosity. Tailoring your hair care routine to these characteristics will help you address issues like dryness, frizz, or breakage effectively.

Ingredients For Healthy Hair

Incorporating the right ingredients into your hair care routine can transform the health of your hair. Essential oils such as lavender, rosemary, and peppermint can stimulate hair growth and improve scalp health. These oils also help balance the scalp's oil production and soothe any irritation. Carrier oils like coconut, argan, and jojoba are excellent for moisturizing and nourishing the hair, adding shine, and reducing frizz. Coconut oil is particularly effective in penetrating the hair shaft and preventing protein loss.

Herbs such as nettle, chamomile, and hibiscus can be used in hair rinses to strengthen and condition the hair. Nettle, rich in vitamins and minerals, helps combat dandruff and promotes healthy hair growth. Chamomile adds natural highlights and soothes the scalp, while hibiscus strengthens hair and prevents premature graying. Proteins, like those from eggs or yogurt, are also essential for repairing and strengthening hair. They help rebuild the hair's structure, making it more resilient and less prone to damage.

DIY Recipes For Shampoos And Conditioners

Creating your shampoos and conditioners is both rewarding and customizable. For a simple DIY shampoo, combine 1 cup of water with 1/4 cup of liquid castile soap. Add a tablespoon of your favorite carrier oil and a few drops of essential oils. Mix well and apply to wet hair, massaging into the scalp before rinsing thoroughly. This formula cleanses without stripping natural oils, leaving your hair fresh and healthy.

For a conditioning treatment, mix 1/2 cup of plain yogurt with 2 tablespoons of honey and 1 tablespoon of olive oil. Apply this mixture to damp hair, focusing on the ends. Leave it on for 20-30 minutes before rinsing out with warm water. The yogurt provides proteins and probiotics, while honey and olive oil deeply moisturize and condition your hair.

Another effective conditioner can be made by blending 1/2 avocado with 2 tablespoons of coconut oil and 1 tablespoon of honey. This rich blend nourishes and smooths hair, leaving it soft and manageable.

Tips For Natural Hair Treatments And Masks

Natural hair treatments can be tailored to address specific hair concerns. For a deep conditioning mask, combine 1/2 cup of mashed banana with 2 tablespoons of coconut oil and 1 tablespoon of honey. Apply the mask to damp hair, cover it with a shower cap, and leave it on for 30 minutes before rinsing. This treatment provides intense hydration and improves elasticity, reducing breakage and split ends.

To combat dandruff and itchy scalp, try a soothing scalp treatment made from 2 tablespoons of apple cider vinegar mixed with 1/4 cup of water and a few drops of tea tree oil. Massage this mixture into your scalp, leave it on for 10-15 minutes, and then rinse with warm water. The vinegar balances the scalp's pH, while tea tree oil has antifungal properties that help reduce dandruff.

Storing And Using Homemade Hair Products

Proper storage of homemade hair products ensures they remain effective and safe to use. Store shampoos and conditioners in clean, airtight containers to prevent contamination. Glass bottles or jars with tight-fitting lids work well for this purpose. Keep your products in a cool, dark place to extend their shelf life and maintain their potency. Homemade hair treatments and masks should ideally be used within a few weeks, as they lack preservatives.

When using your homemade products, apply them as you would store-bought items. For shampoos, use a small amount, lather, and rinse thoroughly. Conditioners should be applied primarily to the ends of your hair, avoiding the scalp to prevent excess oil buildup. For masks and treatments, follow the recommended application times and rinse thoroughly to remove all residues. By following these practices, you can ensure that your natural hair care routine remains effective and enjoyable.

CHAPTER TEN

Packaging And Labeling Your Products

Importance Of Proper Packaging

Proper packaging is crucial in the world of skincare products, not just for aesthetic appeal but also for maintaining product integrity and safety. Effective packaging protects your products from contamination, extends shelf life, and ensures that the ingredients remain effective until use. For beginners, it's important to choose packaging that aligns with your product's formulation and usage. For instance, products with natural preservatives might need airtight containers to prevent spoilage, while products with essential oils might require dark bottles to protect against light degradation.

When selecting packaging, consider factors like the type of product (creams, oils, serums), the storage conditions it requires, and how it will be used by the consumer. For example, a pump dispenser can be ideal for a lotion to ensure easy application and minimize exposure to air. Additionally, proper sealing mechanisms are important to prevent leaks and spills. Testing different packaging options to find what best preserves your product's quality and meets consumer expectations is key.

Eco-Friendly Packaging Options

As awareness of environmental issues grows, many consumers prefer products with eco-friendly packaging. Using sustainable packaging not only appeals to environmentally conscious customers but also reduces your environmental footprint. There are several options for eco-friendly packaging that beginners can consider.

Recyclable Materials: Choose packaging made from recyclable materials such as glass, aluminum, or certain plastics labeled with recycling codes. Glass is an excellent option for many skincare products because it is reusable and can be recycled indefinitely without losing quality. Aluminum tubes or jars are lightweight and also recyclable, providing a durable alternative to plastic.

Biodegradable Materials: Biodegradable packaging materials, like those made from plant-based sources (e.g., cornstarch or sugarcane), break down more quickly than traditional plastics. These materials decompose into non-toxic substances, reducing landfill waste. For instance, compostable bags and containers can be a good choice for products that are intended to have a minimal environmental impact.

Refillable Containers: Encouraging customers to refill their containers can significantly reduce waste. Offering a refill option for popular products allows customers to reuse their existing containers, reducing the need for new packaging. This approach also fosters customer loyalty by aligning with their values on sustainability.

Designing Effective Labels

Designing effective labels is crucial for attracting customers and conveying essential information about your products. A well-designed label should be both informative and appealing. For beginners, the design process involves understanding what information needs to be communicated and how to present it.

Essential Information: Include the product name, key ingredients, usage instructions, and any warnings or precautions.

For skincare products, it's important to list the main active ingredients and their benefits. Additionally, provide information on how to use the product, including application techniques and recommended frequency.

Visual Appeal: Your label design should be visually appealing to stand out on the shelf. Use colors, fonts, and imagery that reflect your brand's identity and the product's purpose. For example, a natural skincare line might use earthy tones and botanical illustrations to emphasize its organic ingredients.

Consistency and Branding: Consistent labeling across all your products helps build brand recognition. Ensure that your labels have a uniform style that aligns with your brand's visual identity. This includes using the same fonts, colors, and logo placement across all product labels.

Legal Requirements And Labeling Standards

Complying with legal requirements and labeling standards is essential for selling skincare products. Different regions have specific regulations regarding ingredient disclosure, claims, and safety information. For beginners, understanding and adhering to these regulations can be complex but is necessary to avoid legal issues and ensure consumer safety.

Ingredient Listing: Regulations typically require that all ingredients be listed in descending order of prominence. Ensure that the names used for ingredients comply with regulatory standards, such as using INCI (International Nomenclature of Cosmetic Ingredients) names where applicable.

Claims and Warnings: Be cautious about making claims on your labels. Avoid making unsubstantiated claims about the effectiveness or benefits of your products, as this can lead to legal issues. Additionally, include any required warnings or precautions, such as "for external use only" or "avoid contact with eyes," to ensure consumer safety.

Regulatory Compliance: Research the specific labeling requirements for your region. For example, in the U.S., the FDA regulates cosmetics and requires that labels provide certain information. In Europe, compliance with the EU Cosmetics Regulation is necessary. Make sure to stay updated with current regulations and adjust your labels accordingly.

CHAPTER ELEVEN

Tips For Sustainable And Ethical Skincare

Importance Of Sustainability In Skincare

Sustainability in skin care is essential for preserving the environment while delivering effective and safe products. The beauty industry has a significant impact on the planet, from resource extraction to waste generation. By adopting sustainable practices, you help reduce this impact and contribute to a healthier ecosystem. Sustainable skincare focuses on using natural ingredients that are grown without harmful pesticides or synthetic fertilizers, which reduces soil degradation and water pollution.

When making beauty products, consider the entire lifecycle of the product, from ingredient sourcing to packaging. Opt for biodegradable or recyclable materials for packaging to minimize environmental footprint. Furthermore, support brands and practices that prioritize renewable resources and energy-efficient processes. This holistic approach not only benefits the environment but also promotes the use of products that are gentle on your skin and free from harsh chemicals.

Sourcing Ethical Ingredients

Sourcing ethical ingredients involves selecting components that are produced concerning human rights and environmental sustainability. Start by researching suppliers who provide transparency about their sourcing practices. Look for certifications such as Fair Trade, Organic, or Rainforest Alliance, which indicate that the ingredients are cultivated and harvested under ethical conditions.

When purchasing ingredients for your skincare products, prioritize those that are cruelty-free and have been ethically sourced. This means they are produced without exploiting workers or animals. For example, choose organic plant-based oils and extracts that are grown using sustainable farming practices. By doing so, you ensure that your products not only benefit your skin but also support a fair and humane global supply chain.

Reducing Waste In Production

Reducing waste during skincare production is a crucial step towards sustainability. Begin by measuring your ingredients accurately to avoid excess and minimize leftovers. Reuse or recycle containers and packaging whenever possible.

For instance, repurpose jars or bottles for new batches of products or use refillable containers to cut down on single-use plastics.

Incorporate practices like batch production, where you make larger quantities of products less frequently, reducing the frequency of production and associated waste. Additionally, explore methods like upcycling, where you use by-products from one process as inputs for another. For example, coffee grounds from a café could be used in a scrub recipe. This approach not only minimizes waste but also adds a unique touch to your skincare line.

Supporting Fair Trade Practices

Supporting fair trade practices is integral to creating ethical skincare products. Fair trade ensures that the producers of raw materials receive fair wages and work under safe conditions. By choosing fair trade-certified ingredients, you contribute to the economic and social well-being of farming communities.

To incorporate fair trade into your skincare business, seek out suppliers who are committed to fair trade principles. These suppliers will provide products like fair trade shea butter or cocoa butter, ensuring that your formulations are not only high-quality but also ethically sourced. Additionally, consider partnering with organizations that promote fair trade practices to further enhance your impact and build a reputation for ethical responsibility.

Educating Others On Sustainable Beauty

Educating others about sustainable beauty is vital for spreading awareness and promoting ethical practices.

Start by sharing information through your website, social media, and product packaging about the benefits of sustainable and ethical skincare. Provide tips on how consumers can make more eco-friendly choices, such as opting for products with minimal packaging or those made from organic ingredients.

Host workshops or webinars on sustainable beauty practices to engage with your audience directly. This allows you to demonstrate how to create eco-friendly products, share insights on sourcing ethical ingredients, and discuss the importance of reducing waste. By educating others, you help foster a community that values and supports sustainable practices, driving collective efforts toward a more responsible beauty industry.

CONCLUSION

In the journey of creating beauty and organic skincare products, we have explored the intricate dance between nature's purity and the science of skincare. Organic skincare, with its commitment to natural ingredients and sustainable practices, stands as a beacon of health and environmental stewardship in the beauty industry. The culmination of this exploration reveals several key insights that underscore the value and potential of organic skincare products.

Firstly, the efficacy of organic skincare products lies in their reliance on pure, natural ingredients. By avoiding synthetic chemicals and harmful additives, these products harness the inherent power of nature to nourish and rejuvenate the skin. Essential oils, botanical extracts, and natural preservatives not only enhance the effectiveness of skincare routines but also minimize the risk of adverse reactions, making them suitable for sensitive skin types.

Furthermore, organic skincare aligns with a broader commitment to sustainability and ethical practices. The emphasis on organic farming reduces the environmental footprint associated with conventional agriculture, including the use of pesticides and synthetic fertilizers. This shift towards eco-friendly practices supports biodiversity, preserves soil health, and conserves water resources. For consumers, choosing organic skincare means supporting brands that prioritize environmental responsibility and ethical sourcing.

The rise of organic skincare also reflects a growing consumer awareness and demand for transparency in the beauty industry. Modern consumers are increasingly informed and conscious of the ingredients in their products.

They seek out brands that not only deliver results but also adhere to ethical standards and transparent labeling. This trend has led to a more educated market, where consumers are empowered to make choices that align with their values and health goals.

In conclusion, the creation and use of beauty and organic skincare products represent a harmonious blend of nature and science, offering benefits that extend beyond skin deep. By embracing organic principles, we contribute to a healthier planet and a more sustainable future. As the beauty industry continues to evolve, organic skincare stands as a testament to the power of natural ingredients and the importance of ethical practices. It invites consumers to experience the profound impact of nature's gifts, not only on their skin but on the world at large. Embracing organic skincare is more than a

choice—it's a commitment to personal well-being
and global sustainability.

THE END